Memoirs of a Tickling Fetishist

ALICE KENTON

DEDICATION

To everyone, everywhere, in your own little corners,
huddled and afraid.

You are *not* alone.

CONTENTS

INTRODUCTION

There's a deliciousness in surrendering control. It's the foundational appeal to almost any BDSM lifestyle, the giving over of one's freedom to the whims of one's partners. Whether it involves spanking, forced orgasms, or any of thousands of potentials, what you are basically doing is putting another person in control of what happens to you, to elicit a response that surpasses the basic reflex and extends into the sexual. A slap on the bottom may draw out a natural cry of pain from anyone, but from the fetishist this is accompanied by a release of brain chemicals that drive the body to pleasure.

This is what most people think of when they are presented with the concept of a fetish—the lifestyle of pain for pleasure. Which is, perhaps, why tickling is not something that immediately springs to mind when one discusses these lifestyles.

With tickling, you not only are surrendering control of your body to your partners, you are surrendering control of your emotional responses. Without causing an iota of pain, one may use a feather, a swath of fur, a hairbrush, a ball-point pen, or even a simple fingertip, and almost instantaneously have their partner collapsing in hysterical fits of laughter. It is an exquisite form of bodily torture and pleasure; the body being forced to exhibit a reaction of delight despite undergoing natural reflexive responses of attempted flight from the stimulus.

Why this is appealing is not something I can easily answer. Perhaps it is the same need for a power exchange found in all other forms of BDSM, but with an aversion for feeling—or causing—pain. Perhaps it is a need to recapture thrills felt in childhood, when tickling and being tickled was far more common, perhaps because it is far more acceptable, than it is when exhibited by adults.

I do not have an answer. But, perhaps, in reading and understanding my story, you may find one anyway.

1 BECOMING ME

While many tickling fetishists can point back to a specific instance in childhood, a moment of physical contact that sparked their awakening, I cannot attest to having had such a moment. Certainly, I had been tickled on the odd occasion, but I did not experience any of the more ruthless experiences others have had at the hands of siblings, cousins, peers, or even adults. My family was quite conservative, and anything that might be seen as even remotely unbecoming was frowned upon. Anything that might give someone an unseemly thought was something not to be engaged in. "Put nothing evil before thine eye," was often quoted, and was the tenet that dominated my choices of books and television shows. A movie could get by with one curse word and earn an arched eyebrow from my mother. A second, and the show would be turned off.

As might be expected, discussion of anything of a sexual nature was kept to a bare minimum. People got married, had children, and when you were ready you would know how that worked. That was the extent of what I would learn when questioned, and anything I felt that fell outside of those very distinct, very bold lines, was something that had to be evil. When our path crossed with two men holding hands in public, I was quickly and roughly steered away. When I asked about what I had seen, I was told they were 'reprobates.'

I did not know what a 'reprobate' was, but I could tell by my father's tone that it was not something to aspire to be. So, when my thoughts eventually began to steer toward other girls, I knew instinctively that it was something I should reject, push down, and certainly, no matter what, never ever discuss.

When I was eleven, my curiosity began to expand. I was old enough now to bathe myself, and I could no longer leave the bathroom undressed with my father in the house. This gave me a certain amount of freedom, and I eventually used the time, naked, to examine my body in ways I never had before. I had once, a few years prior, been getting dried off from a bath, and had bent over to examine my genitals, pulling one of my labia to one side with a finger. The smack I received from my mother made it clear this was an evil thing, and I did not do it again.

But now in the bathtub, with the door locked, I could wonder: Why was it evil? What was bad about this part of my body?

And, in the course of my explorations, I began to develop the sensations one naturally does when manipulating one's genitals with one's fingers.

I was getting horny.

I did not know the word 'horny.' I certainly did

not know the word 'masturbation' or what it meant. I knew that I was touching an evil place and it was feeling good, and I got the sick sensation that this resulting feeling was also evil and not something to be enjoyed.

But it was enjoyable. Why was it so enjoyable? And what was I doing to cause it?

Not having the words in my vocabulary, due to my insular upbringing, I had to rely on the words I did have.

The closest word I could decide upon was 'tickle.'

I was giving my genitals a tickle.

Tickle, tickle.

I orgasmed, for my first time, with the word 'tickle' repeating in my head. And I was frightened to death. I had done something bad, and I was almost certainly going to Hell for it.

I made two vows right then and there: I would never speak of what had happened, never ask questions about what I had felt.

And I was never, *ever* going to do it again.

I did it again.

And again.

And again.

Eventually, I found that, as I 'tickled' my genitals, my mind would entertain me by playing 'movies' in my head, movies starring me and others, women who would tickle the imaginary me and make her laugh, while the real me tickled my genitals to orgasm after orgasm. It was not long before the imaginary me in these mental movies went from being dressed to being naked, exposing all my ticklish places. My orgasms would be more intense when I imagined these things.

But my mind was not the only thing producing movies that would spark my secret, shameful desires.

1977 saw the release of *Raggedy Ann and Andy: A Musical Adventure.* It was a nice, safe, family-friendly cartoon to which my parents would hold no objection to me watching.

I recall with vivid clarity laying on the living room floor, my chin propped up in my hands as I watched the two rag dolls set off on a rescue adventure, because a snooty little French doll named Babette had fallen in with pirates. The brother and sister made friends along their journey, and eventually found their way to the pirate captain. And as they tried to make their escape, this pirate captain called to his aid the assistance of a giant squid from the ocean depths, who captured the heroes, holding one in each of his many tentacles.

And then, the captain gave his command to the octopus:

"Tickle!"

I forgot how to breathe. My heart was in my throat. My mouth had gone dry. And, as I watched this cartoon—this rather simple animation—that had these toys being tickled by the octopus, all of them laughing helplessly, I became aware that I was pushing my pelvic bone into the floor.

The show could not end quickly enough.

Thankfully, it was near the climax—as well was I—and I went straight to my bath for the night as the credits rolled.

This was a new and frightening experience. Yes, I was frequently imagining scenes of me being tickled when I masturbated, but I was in control. I chose when, as convenience and opportunity allowed. But this—this was the first time something *external* had influenced me, had evoked a reaction and compelled me to act.

In my mind, the octopus began tickling the dolls again. The French doll was replaced with an avatar of myself, naked, and I was helpless and laughing hysterically with them.

I was drenched in sweat when I finished, and quickly rinsed myself with the tub water and dried off. But even after my orgasm, the scene would not leave me, and I lay in bed most of the night, staring at the ceiling in the darkness, thinking of that octopus, those laughing dolls, and wondering what other tickling fantasies might be out there in the world.

2 A WORLD OF ONE

Having tickling fantasies and masturbating to them was an exquisite curse. The orgasms I could give myself to these fantasies were far better than those received with any partner. As I got into my older teens and move on into university, I did of course develop relationships—with other girls, much to the shame and disappointment of my family.

But these relationships were always tenuous, fragile. In retrospect, this should not have been surprising. Relationships are built on trust, and I was keeping a large part of my sexual satisfaction locked up tight, in a thick vault, deep in the dungeon of my mind castle where only I could visit it. Even though I had "come out of the closet," I did not dare to come out of my dungeon. I was still too ashamed of my secret, and afraid of the consequences of someone learning about it.

So, I would fantasize about my favorite tickling scenarios when I was having sex, and as anyone can attest, you can always tell when your partner's mind is somewhere else during those moments that are meant to be the most intimate. I'm almost certain they felt I was pretending they were someone else. In reality, I was fantasizing they were simply *doing* something else, something I dared not ask them to perform, not because I was afraid of how it might feel, but because of the potential of their ridicule or, worse, their disgust.

It was funny thing. Coming out as a lesbian seemed so much easier. Being a lesbian was a known quantity. People knew what that was, had seen it in movies—mainstream movies—and daily television programs.

To be sure, the public at large was also aware of the sexual kink community, thanks to lurid daytime talk shows that would parade them about for cheap ratings. "Sticks and stones may break my bones, but whips and chains excite me," was a common joke, and the leather zipper mask was, if not a common thing, at least a known one. One could mention a good spanking with a nod and a wink.

But as for tickling?

Nobody ever talked about tickling. And if nobody talked about it, then it had to mean that nobody thought of it—at least not in the way that I thought of it. I had convinced myself that, out of the billions of people on the planet, I was unique, and not in a good way. While I had numerous normal interactions with people, and made many friends, at times I was the loneliest girl in the universe.

Or so I believed.

3 THE BOOK, THE MAGAZINE, AND THE VIDEO

One of my many joys in the 80s was walking the malls. This was back when the malls were a varied collection of stores, not just endlessly repetitive outlets for overpriced trendy clothing. Every store was something different: toys, novelties, candles, cookies, cards. There were arcades then, crammed with people dropping quarters into any one of dozens of video games.

And there were bookstores. Actual walk-in-and-browse bookstores, before they were gobbled up by the giant chains.

An avid reader, I could spend hours in these places just looking at the titles, thumbing through the interesting ones, and probably reading far more than I should have without actually making a purchase.

It was during one such weekend foray into the wilds of the paper page forest that I found a book that elevated my tickling interests from a passion to a mission: *The Encyclopedia of Unusual Sex Practices*, by Dr. Brenda Love.

The contents were refreshingly straightforward, given the subject matter. Everything was reference neatly and clinically, without judgment. In true encyclopedic form, Dr. Love presented the word for an activity, then proceeded to explain what that activity meant, how it was used in sexuality, and provided references where one could learn more if that applied.

But could it include tickling?

Part of me was afraid to look. I had long labored under the belief that my secret obsession was unique to me, but with always a flicker of hope that there were others with whom I'd be able to interact. If I looked, and there was no reference to tickling, it would confirm my fears, and truly crush my spirit.

The book shook in my hands as I gently turned the pages toward the back of the contents, into the Ts.

And there it was. Tickling. It was a small entry, but it existed nonetheless, which meant that someone, somewhere, did it enough for Dr. Love to know about it.

The few paragraphs discussed various techniques, including the use for swatches of rabbit fur, which was something I had not envisioned. (I soon after acquired myself several different fur samples, which I maintain for personal use.)

But what truly shook me was the footnotes. These referenced the existence of commercial videos. I particularly recall one referenced co-eds, and the other being titled *Ticklish Senorita*.

It was the equivalent of flying over the North Pole,

looking out, and seeing a candy cane forest around a toy factory. They existed. And if they existed, perhaps I might find them.

I read the entry several more times, letting it soak in that somewhere in the world someone harbored the same feelings as I did.

Arriving home, I took to my room with the local phone book, the big thick one with all the business listings lumped into alphabetical categories. Where did I begin looking? Books? Videos?

Unsurprisingly, it was under Adult Entertainment. The category wasn't a large one, but there were a few listings. I scanned the addresses and tried to picture each location. A handful of them were close enough that, were I to visit, it was possible someone I knew might see my car in the lot. Two of them were just outside of twenty miles from home, however.

I wrote down the names, numbers, and addresses, and worked up the nerve to call them.

That took a couple of weeks.

When I finally could take no more of the tension, I sat down with my crumpled note, smoothed it out on my desk, and picked up the phone. With a deep steadying breath and trembling fingers, I dialed the first number.

The man who answered the phone sounded gruff and jaded. I could picture a world-weary cynic, which I am sure was unfair but perhaps accurate, given the clientele he probably dealt with on a regular basis.

"Hello," I said, my voice catching. "I was calling to see if you had any videos about… tickling."

He cleared his throat, and I was thankful he could not see me blush. I felt microscopic, and under judgment.

"We've got some S&M videos that have some tickling in them," he said. "But nothing that's just that. I don't know anything that is."

I quickly thanked him and hung up, heart pounding. I was disappointed. Yes, he had confirmed that there did exist tickling captured on tape, but I had no interest in sitting through who knows how much other fetish play just to see what might have existed. I did believe he was experienced enough to know his wares, however, and my heart sunk that, at least in my area, the tickling videos Dr. Love had made me aware of were not available.

But I still had a second number to call. I may as well be sure.

I dialed the second number, expecting a repeat of the first one.

These expectations, however, did not prepare me for what happened.

"Thank you for calling. How may we help you?"

The voice belonged to a woman. An older woman. A friendly woman. I felt simultaneously more at ease and yet more nervous than before.

"Hello," I replied timidly. "You probably don't have these, but I'm just wondering if you have anything devoted to tickling."

Without pause or any change of inflection, she answered. "Oh, we have quite a bit of tickling material," she said. "We have trouble keeping it in the store, it's very popular. Are you looking for magazines or videos?"

There were magazines? I thought. But of course, there must be magazines.

"Uh, possibly both," I said.

In retrospect, it could not have been more obvious

that I was out of my depth, a virgin among the whores. She had to have noticed it in my demeanor, even over the phone. "Would you like me to check and see what we have currently available?" she offered.

"If it's not too much trouble," I stammered.

I waited in silence for a short while. Moments later, she was back on the phone. "We have about six different magazines right now," she said pleasantly. "And two videos. Would you like me to hold them for you?"

"Thank you," I said. "No. I'm… several miles out, and won't be able to come there until the next weekend."

"It's not a problem."

"Thank you," I repeated. "I'll see what's available when I come in. Thank you." Yes, I could not say 'Thank you' enough times. My mind was in a fog, having confirmed again that these mythical things not only existed, but I actually had a map to their location.

The next weekend, I made the drive into the city. I was on my guard, as I expected to drive through some of the less-safe neighborhoods to visit a porn store. Again, my expectations were defied. Certainly, it was not a little cottage at the end of a suburban cul-de-sac, but neither was it a seedy shack next to a liquor store with bars on the window.

The establishment ostensibly sold lingerie. And then, just past the lingerie, were toys, lotions, novelties, all of which had uses I could only imagine.

There were feather boas and a duster. I did not buy these, but seeing them here made me smile.

A middle-aged woman came up to me. "Can I help

you find something, honey?" she asked. I recognized her voice as the friendly woman on the phone.

"Thank you, no," I said. "I'm just looking."

She smiled. "There's more in the back of the store," she said. "Magazines and videos. If that's what tickles your fancy."

I shivered. She smiled. "I thought I recognized your voice," she said. "We still have the things you asked about."

Dazedly, I followed her to the back of the store, through a doorway into a room surprisingly larger than I would have expected. There were several VHS tapes along the wall, and islands of magazines in the middle. My eyes took it all in, not knowing where to start.

But I need not have worried. My guide knew exactly where to take me, and drew my attention without saying a word by sweeping her arm toward one section of the wall where, prominently featured, was a VHS tape showing two girls, wearing just panties, on a mattress and holding feathers.

"The magazines are on the other side of this unit," she said tapping the magazine rack we stood by. "Let me know if you need anything, honey."

I nodded. "I will. Thank you."

I circled the magazine rack, scanning the titles. I could not have believed there would exist such a variety. My exposure to the pornographic print world had been limited exclusively to *Playboy*, *Penthouse*, and *Hustler*. One time while on a nature walk, I found discarded issues of *Oui* and *Genesis*, but I had never seen them in stores.

These magazines had less-subtle names to them. *Black Cock. Horny Young Virgins. Big Fuckin' Titties.*

I will give them credit, they told you up front what was behind the covers. There were no mysteries to be had here, even though the magazines were shrink-wrapped in plastic to prevent any attempts at browsing. (Had the bookstore in the mall had thought to do this, I might never have come as far as I had.)

Coming around the other side of the rack, I saw the new titles. They contrasted with the others in their coloration, using pastels of pink that seemed to me to be perfectly appropriate. Like the other magazines, however, they were quite direct with their titles. Tied & Tickled was quite obviously about women in bondage being tickled. Tickled Tarts was more of the same. When I picked them up to gaze longingly at the photos on the covers, I found that the wrapping covered two magazines, back to back, so the covers could be seen.

In my head, I counted what money I had brought. It wasn't enough for everything, and I wanted everything. I wanted it all. The magazines were not overly expensive, but the video was truly the prize, and it was not cheap.

I looked again to the VHS. *Bound, Tickled, Tied* from Home Maid videos, starring Dusty and Amanda Lynn.

At some point, I found myself facing the woman who ran the store. She was behind the counter putting things into a bag, and I was giving her money. I wish I had the opportunity to see her again and thank her for being so nice. This was a moment where I could have become quite traumatized and may have put my life on quite a different path. Her gentleness and pleasantness had a calming effect. I even smiled as I left the store, with my video and a wrapped pair of *Tied & Tickled* and *Tickled Tarts*.

The twenty-plus mile drive home was interminable. The brown paper bag in the passenger seat next to me was the most alluring thing I had encountered up to that point in my life. Its contents were a delicious mystery, calling to me with a siren's promises of pleasure waiting to be released. Had I been wearing something less restrictive than denim jeans, I probably would have touched myself as I drove. I could not wait to get into those magazines.

That's not hyperbole. I literally could not and did not wait. I drove just far enough to find a parking lot with empty spaces enough from foot traffic where I felt I could peruse my pornographic treasure in relative safety.

I slid the double-pack of magazines from the paper sack and started to tug at the plastic overwrap. It was not as easy as all that, as I kept the magazines below the dashboard, below the steering wheel, so my leverage was not the best. But even where I was, I felt I was risking being seen.

The plastic stretched, then ripped. I slid it off the magazines, feeling their slick covers, and discarded the wrap into the passenger floorboard.

As clandestine activities went, it was nerve wracking. My posture was awkward, I could not hold the magazine open fully, and I was peering at it through the gaps in the steering wheel. Every car that drove into the parking lot seemed to go past me first, and I knew they were looking at me, head bowed low, and were aware that I was certainly not praying.

My neck ached from leaning forward to keep the pages hidden. But as awkward as it was, it was also exhilarating. The poses of women, undressing each other, placing themselves in bondage, and then being tickled—or at least posing a simulation of it—was more powerful than anything I had imagined. Yes, it was cheesy; the pictures could have been taken the prior year or ten years earlier, it was hard to tell. I didn't care. It was more validation that I was not alone, and knowing that was just as important as the cry of my libido to get us home where we could watch the contents of the videotape.

I slipped the magazines back into the sack and drove, my body quivering with the anticipation of seeing in action the things my mind had conceived of only in fantasy for so long.

Bound, Tickled, Tied was not going to win any adult video awards for Home Maid or the two actresses. There was no overarching plot to the piece, no themes to be developed, no real story to be told. The two actresses were simply on a couch, before a nondescript background, pretending to watch a movie that had tickling in it. This gives them the idea to try it on each other. A brief cut, and both girls are suddenly nude, one tied to the pull-out sofa while the other begins tickling her.

But I wasn't there to judge quality. Truth be told, I was just like them myself: suddenly naked on a pull-out sofa against the plain white wall of my rented studio apartment, watching in rapt attention, my heart elated at the sound of giggles being forced from the girl who was bound and tickled. Of course, my arousal was already ravenous before I even slipped the tape into the player, because of what the tape represented. Tickling was a thing—an actual sexual thing. And I was seeing it being conducted by two adult women as a sexual thing for the first time in my life.

That first time was the best. The second through fifth times were not so bad either. But with repeated viewings, I began to notice the flaws: the production values, the lack of makeup on the actresses allowing for the visibility of small bruises on their legs, the absence of any soft-lensing of the photography. It was cheaply produced compared to the many lesbian porn films I had watched which were of much higher quality, both in production and conception.

Yes, this video confirmed for me that tickling was a real thing. But it was nevertheless a fringe thing, a rarity among the other types of fetish. This I could tell while in the shop, as there were countless bondage videos and just the one devoted to tickling, innumerable magazines about fetishes, but just the handful of tickling magazines.

I was happy to know it existed, but it was still, to me, 'the desire that dare not speak its name.'

I went back for the other magazines as soon as I could.

4 PROFESSIONAL HELP

While I was not quite a regular at the adult entertainment store, I frequented it enough to browse around the rest of the place. As I had seen before, they did sell items that should have been used for tickling—feather-tipped crops, soft dusters, and the like. But while the intent was obvious, the marketing was missing the boat entirely. None of the imagery actually showed tickling, merely a woman showing a (presumably fake) expression of sexual pleasure. I did not waist my money on these things, intrigued as I was by their purpose. Tickling was not the kind of thing you could perform on yourself[1], so there was no need for such implements.

But there were other things of a non-tickling

---

[1] In fact, I was able to tickle myself, but not for long and only on my feet, which are the hyper-sensitive to being tickled. My implement for this was a potted aloe plant. However, reflex always wins, and I was always forced to stop quickly before I could even laugh.

nature that did capture my interest, especially on those visits where I would find nothing new in the way of tickling material. There were newsletters, locally and nationally produced, catering to swingers and such, people looking for hookups and rendezvous and affairs. These were, of course, sealed on the edge with little white tabs. If you wanted to see who was looking, and for what, you had to pay the price.

One such newsletter promised domination and kink, and, finding nothing to feed my tickle yearnings and not wishing to return empty handed, I picked it up as an impulse buy to peruse later that night. There was no intense need to dig into the contents with this, and I almost forgot about it until I pulled out my bed and settled in.

It was, as I had expected, a cornucopia of different calls for BDSM encounters. Threesomes, watersports—the offers ranged from the banal to the extreme. None of it interested me. But in the back pages there were the advertisements placed by those who did such things professionally. If you needed an escort, you could call a number. If you wanted a dominatrix, there was a number. If you wanted to act out any fetish fantasy…

My fingers traced over the ad. Certainly the woman in the image was just another piece of photographic clip art, not the one actually offering to perform services. I wasn't' that naïve. But did her services include what I was interested in—without adding on all that other unnecessary trappings of other fetishes? Because, at that time, I did not believe other fetishes applied to me. I was interested in tickling, and solely in tickling.

I was soon to learn how much more affected I could be by my fetish if I opened my mind—and saw what was already in it.

Any thoughts I had about how this process worked evaporated when I actually became involved with it.

First, there was the phone call. I explained that I was calling about an advertisement, being very vague about the context of it in case I had dialed a wrong number.

The woman asked if it was the advertisement in a certain newsletter, naming it, so I knew I was talking to the right person.

"Yes," I said. "It stated that you work with all types of fetishes." I found I was just as nervous here as I had been that first time calling the video stores, and perhaps with better reason. I was making an entirely different kind of solicitation here.

"I'm set up for almost everything you could think of," she said. Her voice was friendly, but also business. I got the impression she got a lot of calls asking people to describe what she did, so they could basically get free phone sex.

"Even tickling?" I asked, getting to the point.

"Certainly," she said.

She named a price. It was steep for me on my salary at that time, but within reach. I had received a Christmas bonus that year, and it was well more than what was being asked. I agreed to the price, and we set up a time to meet her at a given address.

It was the longest ten days of my life, or so I thought. The week after that would be even longer, but I did not know that then.

On the morning of the appointed day, I showered and washed my hair. I got dressed. Then I sat and watched the clock. Then I showered again and changed clothes. I had a neurotic need to be absolutely clean for her, as I imagined being naked in front of this stranger.

And that is what I was doing. I was going to be naked to a stranger. What is more, I would likely be in some kind of bondage. What if I were running into a serial killer? I had told no one of my plans. I could not. Surely serial killers did not advertise in fetish magazines? But then, why would they not? A smart wolf finds the sheep who are eager to come to him.

I went anyway.

My nerves were on edge. I knew that at any moment, I would be stripping my clothes off, exposing myself to a woman I had not even seen, probably dressed in leather with a mask and carrying some kind of whip. I pictured her stiletto heels being at least eighteen inches high.

The woman who greeted me was far from that. She wore a flowered blouse and blue jeans. She was, from my estimation, twenty years older than I was at the time, putting her somewhere in her mid-to-late forties, and a few inches shorter than myself. She was the most non-threatening human being I had ever encountered, and was astonishingly...normal.

We sat in her living room, side by side on the couch.

"So you're the young lady who wants to be tickled?" she asked. Her voice was disarmingly pleasant. "Is this something you're very sure about?"

This isn't something I expected. I thought it was to be a cash transaction and then just action. This felt more like a job interview.

"I'm—fairly sure," I stammered.

"Have you ever been tickled before?"

"Of course," I replied.

She raised an eyebrow.

"It's—been a while," I admitted. "Like, twenty years or more."

She nodded. "It's fine if you haven't," she said. "I just don't want to get started on something, then have you wanting to back out. A lot of people think they want something until they actually get it. There are no refunds, by the way."

She asked for the payment. Cash. I handed it to her, and she nodded at the coffee table. I placed it there, then she picked it up. It seemed an odd ritual.

"Why do you want to be tickled?" she asked plainly.

Why? I thought. Why would I not want to be tickled? It was only what I had been craving my entire life. Which is what I told her, spilling my fantasies that I had built up ever since that first one.

"Tell me about that one," she said, as I told her I had developed fantasies when I was younger about being tickled by women. "Do you still feel that way?"

I blinked. "Yes, I've always felt that way," I said.

"And you've revisited the same fantasies ever since?" she asked. "Being tickled by a teacher? A nurse? Your mother?"

I shifted nervously. I sudden felt like I was under a microscope, and I did not like this uncomfortable interrogation.

"I've heard enough," she said, patting my knee as she rose. "Come back next Saturday." She gave a time.

"Next Saturday?" I said. I was taken aback. "I thought—"

"Oh, we can't today," she said. "If you were to pay me today, and then we went off to play games, people might get the wrong idea."

I understood. She was separating the act of the payment from the act of the domination. The distance gave her plausible deniability. My heart sank, as my adrenaline levels crashed. I was to wait another week. "Of course," I said, standing to leave. "Next Saturday."

"See you then, honey," she said, and saw me to the door.

One week later, I was standing again outside her door. Would she even be there? Did she take the money and run? No, it was not enough money to make that kind of a scam worth the while. But what if she just didn't answer the door? What if she denied knowing me? That could happen.

I rang the bell.

She answered, just as unassuming as before, completely normal and completely pleasant.

"There's my little girl," she said cheerily. "Come right in. Mommy's been expecting you."

I felt a lump in my throat. Did she just say what I thought she said? I wondered if she had confused me with one of her other clients. I knew there were people into the age play scene from what I had read, but I had never seen the appeal to it. My core desire was and always had been tickling.

Hadn't it?

I followed her into the house, and started after down her basement steps at her beckoning. "I'm a little nervous about being tickled," I said. This was true, but it was also a gentle reminder as to why I was there, in case she had mixed up clients.

"I'm sure you are, sweetie. Don't you worry about a thing," she said. "Your Mommy will take very good care of you."

The finished basement had been set up into separate rooms to make it feel less like a dungeon. Although, in fact, that is exactly what it was—just a nice carpeted dungeon with dropped ceilings. I could see into the first two room that there were the usual straps and tables and leather tools. I shuddered at the idea of what went on in them.

She went into the third room. I followed, and she closed the door behind us.

The room was slightly different than the others. There was a table which had been covered with a mat and a duvet cover to make it look like a bed. The coverings were pink, with lacy trim. The corners of the table had restraining straps ready to be used, but were covered with pink fur.

There was a lace pillow, pink. Two stuffed animals, both pink. Looking back, it was like the room had been transported out of some twisted Disney Princess version of *Fifty Shades of Grey*.

"I don't understand," I stammered.

She looked me in the eye before proceeding. "You told me in our last chat that you had carried fantasies of being tickled by an adult. Are you also an adult in these fantasies?"

The realization shocked me. "Well—no, but..." It was true, my self-image in those fantasies had remained locked at the age at which I developed the fantasies. "But I don't have those kinds of fantasies.

Except for the ones I said, and that's me, so…"

"Our first fantasies are very primal," she said. "That you've carried these fantasies for so long, unchanged—I think you need to let your inner child have what she's wanting. Now…stand still."

As I stood there, obediently, she began to undo the buttons of my blouse. I didn't know what to do. Should I help? Should I not? But soon enough all my buttons were undone and she was working the snap of my jeans. "Just let Mommy take care of everything."

This was definitely not what I had signed on for. And at the same time, I was insanely aroused. I could not move—I did not *want* to move. What I wanted to do was to stand there and let this woman continue undressing me. And honestly, the way she was doing it, the manner in which I was being treated—it was speaking to something in me that was listening, even as it embarrassed me.

Lost in that fog of thought, I became completely naked, and she took my hand and led me to the bed. My mind numb, my body on fire, I got up onto the prop bed and let her take my wrists and ankles, placing them into the soft fuzzy cuffs. Secured, she took the two stuffed animals and snuggled them against my neck.

It wasn't a reproduction of my own childhood room, but it was nonetheless having the effect of making me feel innocent and childlike. I was captivated. So much was I lost in this swirl of new emotions, I yipped with sharp surprise at the feel of her fingernail on the sole of my left foot.

"Let's find out where my little girl is ticklish," she cooed. She circled my body, probing different places with her finger, making me twitch with every poke and stroke. Not having been tickled in years, I was surprised at how intense the reactions were, and these were just brief touches.

Once she had circled me twice, she took a pink feather duster from where it hung on the wall. She began to circle me again, this time using the duster as a probe. This provoked different reactions. The softness in places that were ticklish to firmer touches shivered, and in the places that did not yield giggles before now delivered them up.

The touch across my nipples made them ache. Across my mound made me gasp.

I was awash in arousal.

"Now, baby girl," she cooed.

I gazed up at her, barely able to focus. But I'll never forget the impact of those three little words she said so sweetly.

"Kitchy kitchy koo."

Her nails grazed my soles. Both feet this time, and not in a probing, prodding way, but in steady up and down scratching strokes. It was like being electrocuted. My body spasmed, but the restraints held fast. I thought I would go insane. And I was laughing—oh, laughing so hard! I could not stop the laughter that poured out of me, as she continued to circle my body, tickling me and babying me with every new approach. For the first time, I *was* that girl in my fantasy, and I *was* being tickled silly and I wanted it to never, ever end.

What the hell was wrong with me?

Plenty, I figured. Perhaps more than I had always assumed.[2]

But there was nothing wrong with that orgasm. It came out of nowhere, and crashed through my body with all the subtlety of a building demolition. And I laughed through the whole thing and beyond. I did not even know what she was doing to cause it beyond the tickling. I don't know if she was feathering my genitals, touching them, vibrating them, or if she had managed to magically make me spontaneously orgasm from the tickling alone. But it was fantastic!

I left in a fog of euphoria, my body completely drained and totally blissed out. It was a moment I would (and still do) relive in my mind countless times.

But I was reminded of something that quickly left me feeling my emptiness and loneliness more poignantly than ever: I had just had a life-altering experience, and there was no one to whom I could tell it.

I had every intention on revisiting my tickle dominatrix as often as possible. But time and finances never aligned. Within the year, I and several of my friends were out of a job and on the market, relocating, having longer commutes, taking lesser salaries. Tickling was a strong need in me, but it did not supplant the more basic requirements of my Maslow's hierarchy. Food and shelter still came first. Fortunately I still had my memories and my magazines; and where they fell short, I had my imagination.

Little did I know a change was already taking place

---

2 In my later roleplays, age play would become a common factor, perhaps because there's such a strong connection between tickling as an activity more commonly connected to childhood.

that was going to alter my life—and the lives of everyone on the planet—forever.

5 OMG: WWW

Believe it or not, the Internet was not always with us. Nor was it as easy to use as it is today. There was no Google. You would go to catalog pages to search for items. Search engines like Ask Jeeves, AltaVista, and Yahoo were revolutionary tools.

My latest place of employment had brought this wonderful tool of technology into our environment, and like most humans, we set out to abuse the privilege in record time.

The Internet-connected computers were set off in a corner, where anyone could leave their desk and look up information, then print it out or remember it as they went back to their cubicle. We pretended every search was for the business, but most times we were just "surfing the World Wide Web," reading the latest news stories, and finding interesting blogs to view.

And porn.

So much porn.

One day I saw a gathering of fellows at the computer, typing, stopping, and laughing it up. So I sauntered over to embarrass them, which almost never worked because they knew that I liked looking at the women as much as they did.

The fact that they covered things up and closed windows quickly was a new experience.

"Oh come on," I said. "Share the love."

The fellow at the keyboard—let's call him "Fred"—actually blushed. "Yeah, we, ah, really don't want to spend the afternoon in HR."

I raised an eyebrow. What in the world could they have been viewing that they thought *I* would take offense to?

"Did she at least have a decent pair of tits?" I teased. "You know I love my girls with a decent pair of tits."

Seeing I was not going to leave, Fred slumped and relented. "Right then," he said. "But let the record show I was coerced by this women into engaging in this depravity. I have witnesses."

We all laughed, and he brought the browser back up.

There were no images, and it took me a moment to grasp what I was looking at.

It was a thing called Usenet, and it was the godmother of all discussion boards. Topics were divided, subdivided, and subdivided again until you were in a very narrowly-defined area for conversing.

The current location on the screen was alt.sex.fetish.diapers.

"See," said Fred. "There's all these grown adults what get off on wearing nappies like they're babies." He laughed, and I laughed along with him. I didn't tell him I was already well-aware of the adult baby fetish through my many perusals of the fetish newsletters and video stores.

"So what did you have to search on to find this little gem," I asked him.

"The usual rubbish," he said. "Actually, the search just got us here." He clicked on the hierarchy, and displayed the contents for alt.sex. There were categories for not just fetish, but also bdsm and stories.

"There's every kind of shite in here," Fred said. "We've been making a game of it. Throw out any random subject, and there's an entry for it. What people get into is crazy."

The boys had thus far found fetishes that even stretched my worldly experience, including sexually related conversations regarding Barbies, clowns, cakes, and body inflation.

I knew what I needed to search on. I knew it existed. But I could not bring it up with everyone gathered around.

I threw out a few random nouns and verbs. A few of them got hits, but I was not really paying attention. I was waiting for the moment when I would have a time that was more private.

That Friday, I planned to work late, which wasn't hard as I had several projects to occupy my time. Working late was a common thing with many of my co-workers, and sometimes we would even let ourselves in on weekends to work in quiet solitude. So my being the last person in the room on a Friday drew a few snarky comments about my sad social life, but beyond that teasing it raised no alarms. Still, even after the room had been emptied, I waited another half hour before moving over to the Internet-enabled computer.

I made my way onto Usenet, then followed the chain from 'alt' to 'sex' to 'fetish.'

And then to 'tickling.' I was not surprised that it had an entry—I would have been shocked, in fact, if it had not. And it was quite an active little group, full of people sharing photos, links to videos, creative little fictional tales, and attempts at making hookups between fellow ticklephiles to either trade videos or have actual tickling encounters.

There was so much to enjoy. While there were plenty of photos, these required copying block and blocks of gibberish, to be pasted together in sequence and then decoded by some archiving / unarchiving program. I would later get a copy of this program and go through the laborious process of putting them together. I had plenty of images already, thanks to my small-but-growing collection of tickling magazines. But as they say, once you've seen one lesbian being tickle-tortured, you need to see the rest of them.

The stories, however, were the most accessible of the materials. I put my personal 3.5-inch floppy into the drive and began to copy-and-paste the stories onto it for future reading at home. Many of these were short, brief fantasies about television characters or the actors who portrayed them. Many of them would have been half their size or smaller if the all-capitalized onomatopoeia of laughter were removed. But there were a good many that were also quite engaging, with a modicum of good writing skills paired with a fresh imagination. I was encountering scenarios I had never conceived, and I was loving all of them.

While Usenet had its uses (if you will pardon the pun), it was a bit clunky to use if you were not technically proficient. I read through the threads regularly, getting to know who the regular players were, and learning to know who shared the best photos and stories. But I did not interact, choosing to remain a 'lurker' of the activity.

But this was only the beginning. Almost overnight, people began to create websites with easy to use chat rooms and discussion forums. The most notable of these was the Tickling Media Forum—or TMF as the regulars would call it.

TMF was a virtual explosion of tickling. The forums had stories, images (actual, not decoded files), videos, links to other tickling sites that shared and sold more of the same—anything a tickle fetishist might want would probably be mentioned in the forums and, if it were not, it could be easily brought up in a new discussion thread.

The website also hosted a real-time chat room, with the capability of private chats. This was the beginnings of a small, tightly-knit community that has since grown into some lifelong friendships. The shared love of the fetish may have been a cornerstone—and an important one—of these relationships, but they flourished and grew in other directions. We got to actually *know* each other, beyond anonymized identities adopted to secretly discuss this secret need that needed to be kept secret.

It was, for me, the culmination of a lifelong quest; to not only know I was not alone in my love of the tickling fetish, and not only to have a place where I could quench my insatiable thirst for images, videos, and stories about it, but above all else, to have others with whom I could engage, to share my own stories, and to finally be able to be my true self, without fear of recrimination or shaming.

I was home.

6 OUTED!

It would be very logical at this point for one to assume that tickling dominated my life. And, indeed, it was a major factor. Nightly fantasies and online chatting were a regular activity. However, that is not all a life could or should be. I had friends. I had hobbies. I watched movies (the regular kind, not the tickling porn ones). I read books.

I had relationships. Yes, normal relationships, just like normal people.

Not having the courage to arrange a meetup with a stranger unless there was a cash transaction involved, I nevertheless has girlfriends. Sometimes there was tickling involved, but it was playful (for her, at least, as I gave up nothing about my fetish). And since that would turn me on so much, they were also brief as we found…other things to do.

I had met a girl. Beth. We were quite happy together, and shared an apartment for a while. She worked days, I worked nights, and we spent the intervening hours sharing meals and kisses. When she was gone, that was my time to turn on my laptop and engage in the pursuit of new ideas to stoke the fires of my tickling passion. I did not consider this cheating, as I had come home more than once to find Beth hunkered over her computer with a sexy bit of porn displayed. We would look at it together, and usually end up making love.

That did not mean I wanted her to walk in on my tickle-surfing sessions, though.

One Saturday, we were both going to be home for the entire weekend, and we had made such plans for it. We were going to go out shopping, have lunch at this cute little café downtown, see the latest film, then come home and see where the evening took us.

I was showering. I take long showers. Because of this, Beth and I had worked out an arrangement that I would always let her shower first on days such as this, else I would use up all the hot water—and the last thing I wanted her doing on our special days was to take a cold shower!

Beth had dressed while I was washing up. I finished, toweled off, then wrapped towels around my body and head before going into our bedroom to dress.

When I entered the doorway, I froze. Beth was at the little worktable we had in the corner. Her finger slowly turned the wheel of the mouse to scroll the page displayed on the computer monitor.

A page full of tickling pictures. Pictures I had seen, and quite recently.

I knew what had happened. I had not wiped out the browser history after my last time alone at the machine. I did that sometimes, if I had had a particularly energetic session and needed to wash up or just pass out. But I was always careful to clear that history before Beth came home, if I did not do it immediately after chats.

I have never felt a heart attack before, but I was almost certain I was having one at the moment. My hands started to shake, my mouth went dry, and my chest tightened so that I could barely breathe.

She must have heard me, because she looked over then. I could tell by the look in her eyes she knew. I was already thinking up a story. *Oh, I meant to show you this. Found it last night by chance. Thought it was cute. Ever seen anything like this before?*

But I could tell it was no use. My secret was out.

I did the only sensible thing I could.

I began to cry.

I do not mean that I teared up. I went into a full-fledged fit of sobbing. I was overcome with this irrational need to apologize to her, to apologize for what I was. I could not even look at her, so I buried my face in my hands.

Somehow she managed to sit me on the edge of our bed, or I would surely have collapse. In my mind, I knew what was to come. The dismay, the ridicule. The break-up, and the telling of all my friends. My life was about to be shattered, and I had no way to keep the pieces together.

Today my only regret is that I unconsciously thought so little of Beth as to believe she would be that person I imagined in my little nightmare.

Beth held me through my panic attack. She dried my tears. Then she asked questions. There was no judgment, no anger—just mild annoyance that I had something so important to my sexual identity that I felt I had to hide from her.

She did not think my fetish was freakish. Unusual, certainly. But she also felt it was quaint. Cute, even.

I was calming down, but only barely, as I stammered out answers to her questions. My body trembled, despite how tightly she held me, as I emptied my soul about how long I had lived with these urges and what I did to satiate them.

As I sniffled, wiping tears away with the back of my hand, Beth took the initiative. My towel was wrapped around me, but my arms and shoulders were bare, and she tried to calm me by running a fingertip along the crease of my underarm.

I started. "What are you doing?" I said, still sniffling.

She kissed my forehead. "I'm trying to get you to stop crying, silly." She poked me again, and my body trembled for an entirely different reason.

She turned me to face her. "You are you," she said. "And I love you. All of you, inside and out." With amazing gentleness, she unwrapped the towel I had around me. "Every ticklish inch of you."

My mind rejected that this was happening. My heart told it to kindly shut the fuck up and let things unfold as they were.

This was different than anything I had experienced. This was not the BDSM tickling of a paid professional, nor the convoluted idea of tickling in some trumped-up online fantasy story. It was the gentlest, most loving tickling I had ever experienced, as Beth explored my body like it was our first time together. I giggled like a schoolgirl in love, my fears forgotten, my tears flowing for an entirely better reason.

Tickling became a regular part of our relationship, as I introduced her to the bondage aspects of it. I did not tickle her, not in that way at least. It was not her thing, and I found out that I was actually okay with that. I tickled her during playful tickle fights, but I would always lose those (with intent). Even though it was not her thing, it turned out that I was her thing, even as she was mine, and what made me happy made her happy. And, she learned, she had quite a vicious little tickling vixen in her, as our relationship deepened. One of her favorite 'tortures' for me would be to tie my feet to the end of the bed and tickle them until she was certain I had masturbated to a climax, often playfully not believing me when I claimed to have orgasmed.

Some years later, we parted ways. It was bittersweet, without acrimony. Our lives were simply taking us different directions, literally, with thousands of miles about to spring up between us. I have seen her on occasion, when our lives intersect, and we hug and kiss, and she will often sneak in a tickle with a wink. I will always love her, and perhaps I will love her again if fate permits.

I have had other relationships since Beth. Some of them I have confided my tickling fetish, while others I did not because I could tell it was not something that would flourish. Even for those whom I did tell, there was an element of risk every time, a nervousness about revealing something so personal and intimate. But it never resulted in the apocalyptic destruction of my world that I had always imagined, and I became more confident and comfortable with myself with every new experience and every new person brought into my confidence.

For my confessions, I was never paraded about on television. I never made the national or even the local headlines. I was never even brought in to be questioned at my place of employment.

For all the fear that had held me back the better part of my life, for all the shame I felt over my urges, and for all the guilt I carried for fantasies enacted only in my head or with another consenting partner, I began to realize I could have saved myself a great amount of anguish and self-pity if only I had realized the truth earlier on: the only one who really cared at all about my secret was me.

APPENDIX: FANTASIES

I've mentioned that I have accumulated many fantasies over my many years of having a tickling fetish. And while I may commit them to writing sometime, I thought I might share the various categories, and let you enjoy building on them as you are so inclined. These can all be played in a one-on-one or, for the more daring, in a many-to-one relationship.

Realistic
(Things you can actually play with another person in a physical roleplay.)

- **Interrogation:** You're a captured spy with intelligence vital to your home. Your captors want it, and they plan to tickle it out of you. (A fun way to play this is to pull a random word from a hat first, then put it away or with a third person, then seeing how long it takes you to give up that information.)

- **Physical Exam:** It's time for that yearly checkup, but your doctor/nurse has probing fingertips and you have some particularly sensitive areas that merit further observation.

- **Babysitter:** When it's bedtime, it's bedtime. But how do you wear out a brat full of energy who won't obey? (Turnabout option: How do you convince the babysitter to let you stay up as late as you want?)

- **Abduction:** You have been captured by someone who has no motive other than hearing you scream—with laughter. This one can be fun if you and your partner have to wrestle to get you into your bonds. Clothing that can be discarded is recommended.

Magical

(Things that are best played via chat; unless you figure out a way to make them work for real—in which case, contact me!)

Alien Invasion: They're coming to enslave the world. And how will they subdue us all while leaving us intact to be subservient to them? You're a captured test subject for them to find out what works, and when they discover the effect of tickling on humans, they catalog every way that this can happen and program their ray guns to send these same signals to the entire nervous systems of a target. Of course, these weapons will need a lot of testing…

Mind Master: The dominant party is a hypnotist

who plants key words into your mind to make you feel invisible feathers or fingers tickling you wherever. You also are made slavish to the dominant, so that you obey suggestions such as taking off your clothes or making parts of your body accessible on command. (Technically, with a skilled hypnotist, this fantasy scenario could fall under Realism. However, it is rather unlikely that you will have such good fortune.)

The Tickle Monster: We've all had the Tickle Monster at some point in our lives. In fantasy, the monster can take any form, from human succubus to furry puppet to velvety vine creature. What it craves is sustenance, and what feeds it is the helpless laughter of a trapped victim!

Games

Tickle play can be more than just roleplaying with your partner(s). You can incorporate into a number of games to make them much more challenging and far more sexy. Here are just a few examples that exist:

Twisted Twister
This is your basic game of Twister—with some twists. First, it is played naked (or in your undergarments for the more shy). Second, a position on the mat has to be held for thirty seconds. These thirty seconds begin when the non-posing players begin feathering the posing players wherever they can reach without touching them otherwise. (It's best to make sure there are at least an equal number of players not currently on the mat.) For more experienced players, consider upping the time limits, or replacing the feather with

another tickling tool.

Ticktionary

You pick a word. You try to make your partner guess the word by drawing pictures that represent the idea. But your drawings are a squiggly mess, because the goal of the other team is to keep you laughing too hard to draw using a feather or brush or even a finger, so long as they don't physically restrict you away from the drawing pad (so no tackling tickles). The opposing can appoint a different tickler for each round or keep the same tickler. And for a truly grueling game, the entire opposing team can engage in the distracting tickles.

Dreaded Dominoes

This is one of my favorites and requires a group of friends.

The requirements are a set of double-six dominoes, placed into a pouch. The pips on the tiles have dual representation:

Pips	Body Part	Minutes
1	Neck	1
2	Underarms	2
3	Ribs and Chest	3
4	Tummy	4
5	Pelvic and Thighs	5
6	Feet	6
BLANK	All Over	No Time Limit

The game begins by determining who will be the first to be tickled. That person is then held down or otherwise restrained but free enough so he or she can reach into the bag and draw out a domino.

The person whose turn it is to be tickled controls the shots by determining how the pips on the domino are interpreted. For example, if she pulls a 5:2 domino, she can opt for having her pelvic area and thighs tickled for 2 minutes, or she may decide that her pelvic area is too ticklish even for that and choose to flip the domino pips, and go for having her underarms tickled for 5 minutes. This tickling can be performed by a person selected by a spinner, random drawing, choice, or it can simply be a free for all involving everyone playing.

The blank tile is the wildcard. The tickled person may choose to be tickled "all over" for the amount of minutes determined by the other pips, or to be tickled on whatever body part corresponds to the pips for as long as the tickler wishes to tickle that spot.

The only time the tickled target loses choice is when a double tile is pulled. A 4:4 domino requires the tummy to be tickled for four minutes; a 6:6 domino demands the feet to be tickled for six minutes.

When the current person to be tickled pulls out the dreaded double-blank, the game is effectively over, as he or she will be tickled all over for as long as the party wishes.

ABOUT THE AUTHOR

Hello.

Thank you for reading my story.

My name is Alice Kenton, and I've been a tickle fetishist for most of my life. I've been active in the online tickling community off and on in different guises, and I understand what it's like to live your life in perpetual secrecy.

My hope is that my story may help others cope with whatever secrets they may be harboring that prevent them from living their life to the fullest.

I have written several pieces of tickling fetish fiction, some of which I may actually release some day.

Live your life free of fear.

Laugh.